Chakras For Beginners Ultimate Guide!

Chakras

I0420318

How To Balance Chakras, Activate Chakra Healing, Strengthen Aura And Radiate Energy!

Mia Conrad

STOP!!! Before you read any further....Would you like to know the secrets of becoming a meditation expert?

If your answer is YES, YES PICK ME you are not alone. Thousands of people are learning the incredible benefits of meditation and how it can help you gain control in your mental and physical life.

If you have been searching for these answers for gaining better understanding about meditation and the secrets to mastering this skill, you have stumbled upon the right place!

Not only will you gain incredible insight in this book, but because I want to make sure to give you as much value as possible, right now you can get full **100% FREE access to a VIP bonus Ebook** on the **Secrets of Becoming A Meditation Expert in 7 Days or Less!**

Just Go Here For Free Instant Access:

www.MeditateMind.com

Legal Notice

Disclaimer Notice

information contained herein on the new conditions whenever they see applicable.

Table Of Contents

Introduction

I want to thank you and congratulate you for purchasing the book **Chakras: How To Balance Chakras, Activate Chakra Healing, Strengthen Aura And Radiate Energy!** This compendium is a product of the growing curiosity and public interest about Chakra. It is everywhere – in pop culture, in the movies, and in daily conversations. But what exactly is it? It is the highest hope of the author to somewhat clarify the concepts behind the cool stuff being presented in movies, novels, and anime series.

There are five interesting chapters included in this book. It will be your best and the most practical way to be well-versed with the Chakras. The discussion will involve definition, citing of important situations and examples, and the different classifications of chakras that you should know of. Towards the end, you will be introduced with the concept of mantras.

Hopefully, you will enjoy this introductory discussion. After reading this book, you will be better prepared for higher level of discussions. Additionally, you will find out that after knowing more about chakras, you will be better prepared in using the concepts in actual situations.

Good luck and have fun learning more about Chakras!

Thanks again for purchasing this book, I hope you enjoy it!

Chapter 1 – Chakras For Beginners

Chakra's origin can be traced from Sanskrit. It literally means wheel or vortex. So that explains the usual depiction of chakras in your favorite anime series. Furthermore, experts define it as the center of energy. Ultimately, human beings' consciousness and power are believed to be produced in here.

It has been established that there are seven main center of energy in our body. These points are where the chakra energy is believed to dwell. These energy centers work very much like power plants – they regulate the flow of energy and they mimic the function of pump valves to control the distribution of energy to different systems of the body.

Chakra experts say that one way of knowing how the chakras function for a certain individual is to look at how he is living his life. Depending on the kind of lifestyle that he has is the means by which this powerful energy form is being used. Additionally, chakra distribution is a great way to determine how a person makes his decisions.

And chakra is believed to go beyond the physical. Its influence dwells on the realm of the metaphysical and it stays within the range of the individual's subconscious. It is comparable to an aura, but only the fact that chakra is a lot denser than the aura. Compared to our physical attributes, of course, there is no doubt that the chakra is truly less dense.

But is it, in anyway, similar to the chakra being depicted in the movies, novels, and anime series? For the most part, which might increase your level of excitement and anticipation, the answer is yes. The depictions are accurate as far as the way it is shown to interact with the physical attributes of an individual. If you are wondering through which channel the chakras are being manifested, the answer is through the nervous system and the endocrine system.

Later on in this book, you will find out that there are seven chakras. For beginners, it might be difficult to memorize all of them. But if you are looking for a hint, it would be easier if you know your endocrine glands. All seven glands, except one – the plexus – correspond to a chakra center. The function of each chakra center, as you will find out later, correspond to the function of the gland they are located in.

More importantly all, our perceptions, level of awareness, and sense of being can be rooted to the chakra centers. Therefore, it is a lot more than what you think. In fact, chakras are actually the means to make the impossible a reality.

Chakra – A Closer Look at its History

In case you are wondering where exactly the idea of chakra originated, here is an attempt to trace back its long history. There are many historians who are saying that the word "chakra" is older than the notion of history itself. But it is important to note that the concept, the types, and the hierarchy of the chakra were popularized during the eighth century. Hevajra Tantr and

Caryagiti are said to be responsible to the popularity of chakras and it was during that time when people became a bit more aware of the chakras, its importance, and its manifestations.

The chakras served as the first "hints" that humans have a "subtle body" that lies within the physical body. This "subtle body" is otherwise known nowadays as the soul or the spirit.

India is believed to be the origin of the chakras. This was used in the practice of Ayurveda, a field of traditional medicine. The first time the term chakra was used was believed to be in 2,500 BC. It was used in Ayurvedic medicine because Ayurveda is commonly taken as a body of knowledge that deals with the creation of a sense of balance within a person. Based on the Ayurvedic principles, diseases and sickness can only be corrected through balancing acts like physical exercise, use of herbal medication, and different kinds of meditation. The other major belief of Ayurveda is that the most effective means to achieve healing and wellness is through the manipulation of the chakras – be it via realignment, unblocking, or achieving balance.

The historical conception of chakra is no different from our modern depictions that are shown via pop culture. They are actually seen as circulating energies that are capable of flowing freely. Drawing the link between the body, soul, and mind is only made possible because of chakra channels. Experts say that an individual can only master his chakra control if he has a well-balanced physical, spiritual, and mental health. Ayurvedic medicine would also assure you that there are several hundreds of minor chakra channels in the body, but you only need to focus on the seven major chakras.

Characteristics of the Chakras

Ancient texts would describe chakra according to the categories or type where they belong to. But these ancient texts would also describe the common characteristics of chakras. Here are the characteristics mentioned in these discussions:

*) Though there are no physical representations, chakras are parts of the body. They cannot be removed. Without them, you are incomplete.

*) Locating the chakra is easy. There is a need for you to locate exactly where the channels are.

*) Visually speaking, the chakras are not just round or wheel-like. They also appear to have petals or spokes.

*) There are pairs of sides that tend to sandwich each channel of the chakra. These depict the positions of the chakra.

*) Chakras have colors. There are chakras that are associated with Gods and deities. Finally, they can help in communicating specific mantras.

Chapter 2 – How To Balance Chakras

Achieving a well-balanced chakra system has many benefits, experts say. While there are many others who take this aspect for granted, it should be established that the benefits of balancing one's chakras can go beyond the physical. It can even affect the way a person handles his finances, his health, his dreams and aspirations, and even his future. Therefore, if you wish to achieve success, then you have to know how to balance chakras.

Anyone should have the proper working knowledge about the different variations of energies that can be used and utilized for different activities. From this knowledge, one will know how to use the energies and how to allocate them accordingly.

First, you need to understand that finances are actually controlled by the root chakra. The financial aspect therefore is an essential type of knowledge. Though there are many energies managed in the root chakra, one has to give due attention to this chakra if he wishes to be rich.

At the base of the chakra, one can find the capability to produce. One has to fight off all negative energies in this particular chakra and avoid blockages. By achieving that state of balance, one can commence his journey to become really rich.

Additionally, more than increasing the abundance of material resources, one should understand that chakras also have a great effect on the manner of enjoyment and achieving success. But first, one has to genuinely believe before such changes will be achieved. It is similar to sowing some seeds. Without the symbolic seed sowing process, your chakras won't be aware of the true intentions of the heart and the soul.

Also, the root chakra is not labeled "root" for nothing. Just like a plant's root, it is the chakra from which all other energies originate. By keeping this healthy and open, and by preventing it from being clogged, one has to take care of the root chakra.

Techniques in Balancing the Chakra – the Easiest Ways

Truth be told, balancing the chakra might not be that difficult. Two buzzwords should come to mind: visualization and of course, meditation. These are two of the most common and the easiest ways of maintaining chakras that are prone to being clogged.

Experts say that one has to "feel the chakra" in order to be successful in connecting them with the other chakras. Without "feeling the chakra," it would be impossible to balance them. To make this process simpler to understand and to do, keep the following things in mind:

(*) First, try to do some grounding. Plug up to the elements and feel the earth. The earth still is and always will be the best source of all of our energies.

(*) Do your breathing properly. With proper breathing, anyone can find it easier to make the energy flow from one chakra to another. Proper breathing will help you become more relaxed and by doing so, you will learn the correct chakra route.

(*) Be the master of visualization. It might not be possible for you to see what's happening in your system, but you can clearly see what you want to happen in your life. By visualizing your goals and aspirations, the energy tends to fall into its proper place.

Chapter 3 – Activate Chakra Healing

In this chapter, you will have a better idea on where each chakra is stationed in relation to your physical attributes. By knowing these, one will know how to activate chakra healing. Each of the seven chakras are capable of address different concerns. This will help you accomplish one important task – activate chakra healing. The centers of the chakras should be known because this is an essential step for you to control the flow of energy.

There are also instances wherein you might find your chakras blocked or congested. This is usually the result of lengthy exposure to stress and emotional factors like problems, stress, confusion, and other physiological irregularities. The blockage and congestion can lead to more serious conditions because the energy can be trapped. When this happens, the body parts that are deprived of the energy may not function fully and normally. In the process, not only the body parts will suffer but also the spiritual and emotional aspects as well.

This chapter promises to deliver information about the seven systems of the chakra in a human body:

First System of Chakra: The Base or Root Chakra System

Associated color to this system of chakra is red. It is found at the base or the root of one's body: at the tail end of the spinal cord. Compared to all other systems of the chakra, the base or root chakra system is the most proximate to the ground. Basically, the role of this system is related to that: it is used to constantly be grounded to the earth. It also gives a person the instinct to survive despite physical obstacles or limitation. The body parts that correspond to this system are the following: the feet, the legs, the bones, the large intestines, and the adrenal glands. The first system of the chakra enhances a person's capability to sense whether the better option is flight or fight. If the first system of the chakra or the base or root chakra system is blocked, it can lead to paranoia, procrastination, defensiveness, and fearfulness.

Second System of Chakra: The Sacral or Navel Chakra System

In this chakra system, the color that is associated is orange. The location of the second system of this chakra is in between the navel and the spinal column. Therefore, the organs and systems connected to this chakra system are the following: the kidneys, the bladder, the circulatory system, the lower part of the abdomen, and the reproductive system. The activities connected to this system of chakra are the following: reproduction, procreation, sexuality, creativity, pleasure, and desire. If this system is blocked or clogged, there is a great chance for a person to have problems in dealing with their emotions, especially those connected with guilt in sexual activities, compulsive and obsessive behaviors, and emotional problems.

Third System of Chakra: The Solar Plexus Chakra System

The color that is associated with this chakra system is yellow. It is positioned just above the navel. Usually, it is associated with an individuals' capability to digest the food taken into the system. The body organs and systems that are connected to this chakra system are the following: pancreas, adrenal glands, and different kinds of muscles. According to experts, the third chakra system is the center of a person's emotions. You can never feel happiness, anger, joy, and even power without this chakra system. More often than not, this chakra system stores sensitivity, ability, and ambition. Once the solar plexus chakra system is blocked, a person might feel helpless to the point of being victimized, have the lack of direction, anger, and frustration.

Fourth System of Chakra: The Heart Chakra System

Green is the most commonly associated color with this. This can be located at the very core of a person's heart. This chakra is known for being at the very heart of love, compassion, peace, and harmony. Most of the believers of the chakra system believe that our very soul is enclosed in this particular chakra. There are different parts of the body that are connected to this chakra – they are the thymus, heart, lungs, and the upper extremities. Many people associate the act of finding one's soul mate or life partner to this specific chakra. Also, our capacity to show and feel "unconditional love" is attributed to this chakra system. This is also the center of all our emotions. It helps us feel the signal that we already have to form respective families or to settle down. If this particular chakra is very weak, one may have a weak heart or unhealthy lungs. Also, weakness in the heart chakra will lead to the lack of compassion and love, immoral thoughts and lack of principled actions, and the absence of sense of humanities.

Fifth System of Chakra: The Throat Chakra

Turquoise is the associated color to the throat chakra system. It is located in – yes, you guessed it right – the throat. It is often where our capability to communicate, to express, to create, and to judge are connected. The body parts that are usually associated with this chakra are the following: the hands, the neck, the shoulders, the parathyroid glands, and the thyroid glands. Gaining control mastery of this chakra assists in the proper development of both the skill of inner and outer hearing. The process of purifying or filtering thoughts is also connected to this chakra. It helps in healing diseases and illnesses. It also assists in doing the following: synthesizing information and other kinds of ideas and transforming one entity into another form. Finally, having a problematic throat chakra can lead to miscommunication, capability of saying false words, and the absence of creativity.

Sixth System of Chakra: The Chakra of the Third Eye

By far, this is the most popular chakra because it is often depicted (in a very negative manner) by the pop culture. It is seen in the movies and TV shows. Usually, indigo is the color associated with it. If you wish to locate your third eye chakra, it is at the center of the forehead and aligned with the two other eyes. It is very powerful due to the fact that it is the window towards transacting directly in the spiritual world. Usually, the capabilities attributed to this chakra are as follows: the capacity to ask, to perceive, and to know. The ideals connected to this chakra are the following: intuition, wisdom, and vision. This particular chakra is said to store the best memories, recollections, and even one's dreams and aspirations. If it is blocked, a person is expected to lack foresight. He may also have problems in selecting memories. He might as well experience depression, forgetfulness and difficulty in having flexibility of thought.

Seventh System of Chakra: The Crown Chakra

Violet is the color of the crown. It is on top of one's head. The cerebral cortex, the central nervous system, and even the pituitary glands are all associated with the crown chakra. Its main concern is to properly receive and accurately process all sorts of information, to have a deeper level of knowledge and understanding, to have a sense of blissfulness, and to gain the acceptable level of acceptance. The crown chakra is said to be every person's channel to God or to the Divine Being. Other experts call it as the Divine Purpose's Chakra. If this chakra is blocked, it can lead to insanity and instability of all psychological attributes.

Chapter 4 – Strengthen Aura

Aura is comparable to a bright light or halo that covers not just the head but the rest of the body. It is an approximation of a person's mental, emotional, spiritual, and physical energies.

More often than not, aura comes in different color spectra. They are often associated with color frequency and intensity. The vibration of the aura is usually really fine and really subtle. This needs a high level of sophistication and intuition. It is usually an indicator of what a person can do and what a person cannot do. that is why a person needs to strengthen his aura to do better.

Up until today, fields of science can still offer not exacting explanation for the existence of aura. But if you wish to be very scientific, you will not be disappointed either. If you are aware of the methods of measuring different forms of energy, then you will see a close and deep association between and among these energy forms.

Nowadays, even the field of medicine and other hard sciences use aura for diagnosis. Even medical practitioners are convinced that a person's level of health can be based on a person's aura.

In order to keep a very healthy aura, one should focus on pranic forces. The prana refers to the inner energy that is necessary for balancing astral, mental, emotional, and spiritual health.

Chapter 5 – Radiate Energy For Healing

If you wish to radiate the right kind of energy for healing, then you must read further.

It is no secret that the sun is the ultimate source of energy on earth. Without it, majority of life forms on earth would be impossible. From there, you know that the first form of energy that reaches the earth is in the form of light. And light can be divided further to different colors that represent different energies – ROYGBIV or red, orange, green, blue, indigo, and violet.

Light and color, in effect are not separable. When one knows the represented energy of each color, then one will have a mastery of the different kinds of energy that is radiated.

Why the Chakra System is Important in Radiating Energy for Healing

While not much is understood about chakra, it has been proven that by mastering this aspect of a person's being, a person will have a working knowledge on purging out impurities and toxins. These are the forms of pollution that causes illnesses.

By knowing more about the chakra system, you will have more knowledge about the entire body.

Chapter 6 - Kundalani

Kundalani is a branch of yoga that focuses mainly on awareness. According to experts, this is a very powerful tool known for being truly dynamic and it can enhance the soul's level of experience.

The energy flow is focused on one's nervous system. This way, the physical and mental processes are enhanced. The elements that are usually combined are the following, focus of the eye, locks of the body, posture, balance, lung expansion, pattern of breathing, and blood purification. This way, a better body can result which is essential for a better mind.

Note that the Kundalani yoga is far from being a religion. It is just a process of purifying the body to enhance mental functions and to uplift the spirituality of the person. It is universal. It holds no restriction at all. It does not have to be about religion or denomination.

Kundalani is for people who can deal with daily problems, challenges, and stresses. It can be for housemakers, laborers, students, managers, writers, or health practitioners. It is an open option for everyone. It can help challenge the changing pace of the times.

In the past, Kundalani is a secret kind of yoga. This was the trend until a popular yogi taught this kind of yoga so that more people will be able to benefit from it.

Chapter 7 – Meditation For Beginners

Meditation for beginners – this is where everyone should begin. Meditation is one approach to train a person's mind. If the body needs the gym to tone up, the mind needs meditation. There are many techniques that exist.

In this chapter, you will be given an overview of the different methods of meditation deemed best for beginners:

Technique #1: Concentration Meditation

This enables the meditator to focus on one chosen point. Here, a person may choose to watch his own breathing or repeating a chant in his mind. Others prefer staring at an object or listening to a repeated or periodic sound. There are a few who chooses to count small objects (e.g. rosary beads).

Technique #2: Mindfulness Meditation

Wandering thoughts are shot down through mindfulness meditation. This way, he can travel into his own thoughts. No, the intent is not to judge the person, but to increase his level of awareness when it comes to what comes in and comes out of his mind. By doing this, thought patterns can be drawn.

Other Techniques for Meditation for Beginners

Compassion cultivation is one technique that is very simple yet very noble. It is a practice that is done on a day-to-day basis by Buddhist monks. This involves the process of envisioning negative effects of events and remodeling such so that they can become more acceptable and the transformation can only be possible if you know how to use your compassion. Others use kung fu, tai chi, and even meditation through walking as techniques for beginners.

Benefits that Can Be Derived from Meditation

Note that if you think that relaxation is the ultimate goal of meditation, then you are getting it wrong. It is merely one of the tangential effects of meditation. The following are some of the benefits that may be derived from meditation:

(*) lower level of blood pressure

(*) better quality of blood circulation

(*) marked improvement and normalization of heart rate

(*) lower level of perspiration

(*) acceptable level of respiration

(*) less fear and anxiety

(*) lower level of cortisol in blood

(*) greater feeling connected to the betterment of well-being

(*) lower level of stress

(*) deeper level of relaxation

If you are still wondering how meditation should be done, then you might be interested in doing the following steps:

(*) First, find a spot where you can lie down or sit comfortably. There are many people who purchase a chair that is made especially for meditation.

(*) Next, the eyes should be kept shut.

(*) No effort should be done to control or restrain your breath. It is always better to do the natural way of doing breathing.

(*) The attention should be placed on breathing. The process of inhalation and exhalation should be normalized. The chest, belly, rib cage, and even the shoulders should be kept under close watch.

Chapter 8 - Mantras

Mantra is a word that literally means "mind instrument." Therefore, this can pertain to the powerful energy or vibration that is usually used as a pace setter or rhythm for meditation. In this particular chapter, some important concepts about mantras will be tackled.

According to the traditional Vedic definition, it is important to have proper discernment and discrimination of different kinds of sounds that are naturally-occurring. To illustrate, each sounds from nature have specific vibrations. For example, we have the wind, animals, thunders, rivers, and even the insects. Each sound manifests the kind of soul that each creature possesses.

During the ancient times, the clairvoyant members of the communities rely on their mantras in making their predictions. Healers also use these in carrying out their roles. Subsequently, given these important roles of mantras, they found a special spot in the history of the Vedas.

Technically, mantra stands for holy utterances. It can be a syllable or a sound that can be represented by a phoneme. According to experts, such mantra has a great effect on the power of a person's spirit. Mantra can go beyond syllables. They can also be in form of words or phrases. More than what can be heard, the mantra should likewise be manifested in a person's level of consciousness and even in their thoughts and deeds.

It was during the early Vedic era when people first thought of recording (through writing) the different kinds of mantras that were used in their different ceremonies, rituals, and rites. In approximation, the records are already three thousand years old already.

Depending on the philosophy or school of thought, the mantra has different use, function, significance, structure, and importance. Also, there are different kinds of mantras that can be classified depending on their forms. Usually, they can be sung even by ordinary people. That's where the appeal comes in. Aside from the appeal, it also communicates the concepts of truth, action, reality, knowledge, peace, immortality, light, and love. But what can be understood best is the fact that mantras are meant to actually lift our spirits.

Centuries ago, Renou proposed that mantra is just a plain thought. But later, it was qualified that mantra is more than that. While it can be classified as thought, it is a higher form of thought.

Chapter 9 – Different Chakra Mudras

Yoga and tai-chi are two of some exercise forms that have been rediscovered and are currently peaking in terms of popularity. These two forms of exercise that do not merely focus on the physical aspects give due importance to psychological, mental, and spiritual aspects of a person. While there are many people who would dismiss these exercises as mere venues to display their physical skills, it should be noted that it goes beyond that. Truth be told, there are many mudras that help out in tapping the maximum potentials of the chakras. They are especially useful for meditation.

Mudras can be defined as gestures with specific meaning that are often adopted for enhancing meditation. Mudras are helpful in channeling energy to different parts of the body. The following are the different Chakra Mudras:

The Gyan Mudra

This is commonly known as the mudra of knowledge and is believed to assist in obtaining a fresh mind. In order to do this mudra, one has to let his index finger touch the tip of the thumb. For the remaining fingers, they should be extended in the most relaxed manner possible.

The Vayu Mudra

The good thing about this mudra is that this can be done while you are standing up, sitting down, or when you are resting while lying down. The index finger has to be folded and the phalanx bones should be a bit visible. Once the finger is folded, the thumb should press on the bone. All other fingers, on the other hand should be relaxed and extended.

The Agni Mudra

This mudra is often associated with the element of fire. By folding one's ring finger, this mudra can be achieved. The folded finger's middle bone should be able to press the base of the thumb. Again, all other fingers should be extending outwards. This brings the best results if done in upon waking up and sitting down. Experts say that one can do this best with an empty stomach. To see significant effects, this has to be done for 15 minutes every single day.

The Prithvi Mudra

This mudra is associated with the earth element. To be able to do this, the tip of the ring finger should be able to touch the tip of the thumb. The tips of these fingers should press each other really well with the other fingers extended really well. This can be done at any time within the day, but it is often recommended to do this in the morning.

The Varun Mudra

This mudra is best associated with the water element. This is known to invite positive mood. This can effectively eliminate stress from your system. The little finger's tips should press the thumb's tip. The other fingers in between should be kept straight yet relaxed.

Chapter 10 – Spirituality And Mindfulness

According to experts, emotional intelligence and other desirable attributes are related directly to spirituality and mindfulness. In fact, these two main points of the chapter are essential in developing a person's development of the sense of self-awareness. Ultimately, reality can be tested through spirituality and mindfulness. Somewhat, this is related to coming up with solutions to many problems and tolerating stress.

A person can only be truly spiritual and mindful through meditation. In an earlier chapter, meditation was fully discussed. If only everyone will have the skill to perceive everything through the lens of meditation, it will be much easier to acquire wisdom. Cultivation of wisdom can only be possible through gaining more experience. This is the only path towards the state of non-judgment and non-expectation.

Doing mindfulness and spiritual meditation

In order to do this successfully, one has to spend time dwelling on the physical – knowing what's going on with aspects connected to the physical. This sense of awareness will make the state of stillness possible. You need to point out all of the sources of discomfort. But you should also answer the question: What makes me feel comfortable at this point? The movement and breathing patterns should be watched out closely, too. Also, all thought trails should be monitored closely. By doing these essential steps, you can bring yourself to a state wherein a higher degree of mindfulness and spirituality can be reached.

Personal and professional aspects also need to be considered when you move into the phase of meditation. Problems, challenges, and sufferings should also be considered. Note that meditation is not a means to escape problems and challenges; it is a means to achieve stability despite these problems and challenges. By considering these important aspects of your being, you can reach a point wherein you are aware of everything.

Are there specific methods of practicing spirituality and mindfulness?

It begins with entering a state of mindful and spiritual meditation. Once it has been reached, you can readily remember that state. By remembering that state, you can easily replicate or reproduce that state of body, mind, and spirit. Therefore, in simple terms, mindfulness and spirituality can only be truly attained via repetition and replication. The ideals that need to be followed are the following: compassion, appreciation, acceptance, and affection.

The state of mindfulness and spirituality can only be truly revealed to you if you embody the ideals mentioned above. These ideals are a bit overwhelming because of the fact that they are too simple. Once the point has been reached, it can be practiced anytime.

Mindfulness and spirituality is only one of the several ways to thoroughly improve a person's point of view in finding the true sense of living. By possessing this sense of awareness, a person can reach the point wherein he is truly in control – of his feelings, thoughts, emotions, and actions. The point of spiritual and mindful equilibrium is equivalent to being awakened.

Conclusion

Thank you again for purchasing this book on **Chakras: How To Balance Chakras, Activate Chakra Healing, Strengthen Aura And Radiate Energy!**

I am extremely excited to pass this information along to you, and I am so happy that you now have read and can hopefully implement these strategies going forward.

I hope this book was able to help you understand the nature of chakras and how to maximize their benefits in our daily lives.

The next step is to get started using this information and to hopefully live a full and happy life!

Please don't be someone who just reads this information and doesn't apply it, the strategies in this book will only benefit you if you use them!

If you know of anyone else that could benefit from the information presented here please inform them of this book.

Finally, if you enjoyed this book and feel it has added value to your life in any way, please take the time to share your thoughts and post a review on Amazon. It'd be greatly appreciated!

Thank you and good luck!

Preview Of:

The Ultimate Spirituality Guide!

<u>Spirituality</u>

Understand Spirituality And Spiritual Growth - Gain Peace Of Mind Using Mindfulness Meditation, Emotional Intelligence, And Other Awareness Techniques!

Introduction

I want to thank you and congratulate you for purchasing the book, *"The Ultimate Spirituality Guide! Understand Spirituality And Spiritual Growth: Gain Peace Of Mind Using Mindfulness Meditation, Emotional Intelligence And Other Awareness Techniques"*.

This book contains proven steps and strategies on how to be mindful and how you can nurture your spiritual growth.

Living a spiritual life can help your be free from unhealthy attachments. It can be easy to get caught up with the erratic flow of the external world. Most of the time, people are concerned about the past or the future that they forget to experience the present moment.

Once you decide to nurture your spiritual growth, being mindful about everything in life can come naturally. Your psychological health and emotional intelligence influence how you deal with life's conditions and how you handle relationships in your life. People can accumulate a lot of pain and regret from the past or hide secret desires and resentment. All of the emotions that settle inside you can prevent you from connecting with your spiritual side.

The spiritual path is a lifelong journey and spiritual transformation does not happen overnight. There are a lot of things that you can do to enhance your spirituality like meditation and being mindful.

As you will learn in this book, meditation enables you to see situations and problems with clarity without providing any judgment or criticism. Practicing mindfulness can help you appreciate the seemingly mundane things in life and help you have an attitude for gratitude. Meditating few minutes a day and reminding yourself to be mindful can greatly help you live a more peaceful and happy life. Start your journey towards spirituality with meditation and the other techniques shares with you in this book.

Thanks again for purchasing this book, I hope you enjoy it!

Chapter 1: What Does Spirituality Mean? Why Is It Important?

Spirituality can be defined as the desire to grow your personal relationship with God or nature. Spirituality is a vision of life for a person. It is not simply composed of beliefs that stay in the head, but rather it gives direction to your ideas and actions.

Developing spirituality is also an ongoing endeavor where you nurture it and practice it for your entire lifetime. Spirituality is oftentimes confused with religion. All religion put emphasis on spirituality as part of their practice but it is possible to be spiritual without being part of a particular religion. Spirituality is more of a personal relationship with God and the desire to make that connection deeper and more developed.

Importance of Spirituality

The benefits of spirituality extend beyond emotional satisfaction. There is a growing body of evidence that also proves that it can be associated with better emotional intelligence and better health.

Contemplative practice is good for people

Contemplative practices are activities that direct your focus to a specific sensation or concept. The practice can also focus in an inward reflection. Many traditions all over the world use these practices to increase their empathy, compassion as well as to have a peace of mind.

Examples of contemplative practices:

- Prayer. Prayer can give a person a feeling of hope, gratitude, and compassion. While there are many types of prayer, all are rooted in a belief that there is a higher power that can influence your life. This belief provides a sense of comfort during difficult times.

- Journaling. Writing your thoughts is a way for you to understand your inner self. Studies show that journaling while experiencing difficult times can help you through life's challenges, making you more resilient to obstacles.
- Meditation. Meditation can induce calmness and concentration. Richard Davidson's research shows that meditation can increase the brain's gray matter density. This can increase pain tolerance and enhance your immune system.
- Yoga. Yoga is an old practice that aims to create a union between the body and mind through postures and breathing expansions. Yoga can reduce stress, depression, and anxiety.

Spirituality can help you make healthier choices

Following a spiritual principle can also have a health benefit since it usually promotes treating the body with respect and avoiding unhealthy behaviors. Research shows that people who are adhering to their spiritual guidance are less likely to commit a crime or be involved with vices.

Helps with mental health problems

Spirituality can help people deal with mental illness and can help a person feel less lonely. Spirituality also gives people mental resilience and enable people to make sense of what they are experiencing.

Teaches people how to forgive

Learning how to forgive enables you to move forward in your life. Whether it is learning to forgive other people or yourself, research shows that forgiveness has numerous health benefits like reduced blood pressure, longer lifespan, and improved cardiovascular health.

Enables you to understand yourself better

Being spiritual enables you to understand yourself better. Some people are able to connect with their inner self through prayer or meditation while others find it in nature or even music. Understanding yourself helps you make sense of your feelings and understand the root cause of your problems.

Find the best things in life

Spirituality helps you appreciate the good things in your life. You can't appreciate anything if you are stressed or angry. Setting aside few minutes to hear the sounds, smell the scents, or see the colors around you can help you get away from stress for few minutes.

Thanks for Previewing My Exciting Book Entitled:

"Spirituality: The Ultimate Spirituality Guide! Understand Spirituality And Spiritual Growth - Gain Peace Of Mind Using Mindfulness Meditation, Emotional Intelligence, And Other Awareness Techniques!"

To purchase this book, simply go to the Amazon Kindle store and simply search:

"SPIRITUALITY"

Then just scroll down until you see my book. You will know it is mine because you will see my name "Mia Conrad" underneath the title.

Alternatively, you can visit my author page on Amazon to see this book and other work I have done. Thanks so much, and please don't forget your free bonuses

DON'T LEAVE YET! - CHECK OUT YOUR FREE BONUSES BELOW!

Free Bonus Offer: Get Free Access To The www.MeditateMind.com VIP Newsletter!

Once you enter your email address you will immediately get free access to this awesome newsletter!

But wait, right now if you join now for free you will also get free access the "Secrets of Becoming A Meditation Expert – In 7 Days!" free Ebook!

To claim both your FREE VIP NEWSLETTER MEMBERSHIP and your FREE BONUS Ebook on the SECRETS OF BECOMING A MEDITATION EXPERT IN 7 DAYS!

Just Go To:

www.MeditateMind.com

www.ingramcontent.com/pod-product-compliance
Lightning Source LLC
Chambersburg PA
CBHW071152280526
45787CB00003B/1496